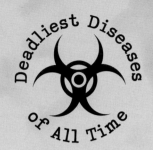

Deadliest Diseases
of All Time

Hepatitis

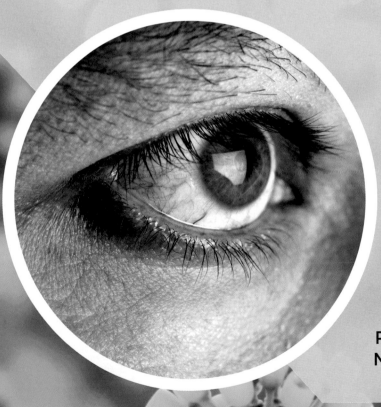

Petra
Miller

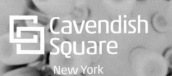

Cavendish
Square
New York

Published in 2016 by Cavendish Square Publishing, LLC
243 5th Avenue, Suite 136, New York, NY 10016

Library of Congress Cataloging-in-Publication Data

Miller, Petra.
Hepatitis / by Petra Miller.
p. cm. — (Deadliest Diseases of All Time)
Includes index.
ISBN 978-1-50260-650-1 (hardcover) ISBN 978-1-50260-651-8 (ebook)
1. Hepatitis — Juvenile literature. 2. Hepatitis — History — Juvenile literature. I. Miller, Petra. II. Title.
RC848.H42 M55 2016
616.3'623—d23

Editorial Director: David McNamara
Editor: Fletcher Doyle
Copy Editor: Cynthia Roby
Art Director: Jeffrey Talbot
Senior Designer: Amy Greenan
Senior Production Manager: Jennifer Ryder-Talbot
Production Editor: Renni Johnson
Photo Researcher: J8 Media

Printed in the United States of America

Contents

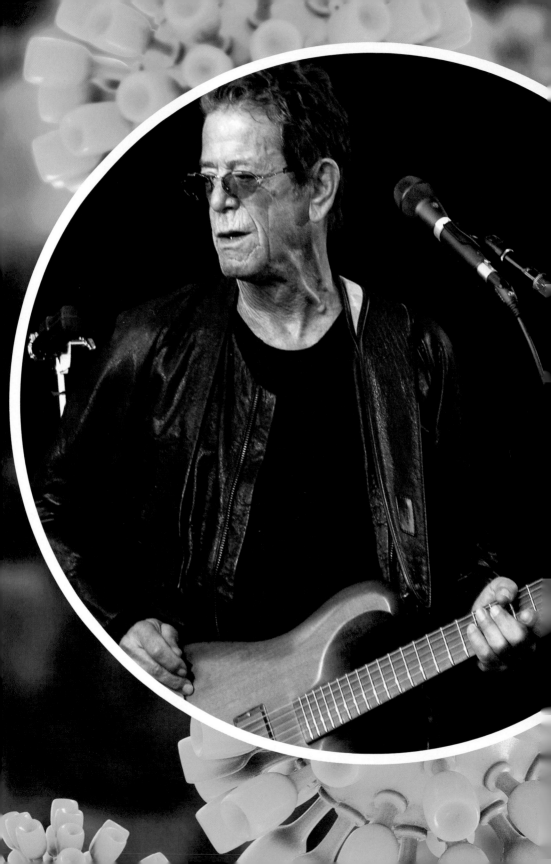

Introduction

Lou Reed was a singer and musician whose influence extended far beyond his work in the 1960s with the band Velvet Underground. His songs were covered by REM, David Bowie, and Nirvana. It is said that the punk, glam, and alternative rock movements of later decades were indebted to him.

Reed had a long career, and for most of it he probably carried one of the world's deadliest diseases. He died of **liver** failure in October of 2013, after a long battle with hepatitis C. He probably **contracted** the disease from intravenous drug use, which is a common method for spreading hepatitis.

People with hepatitis can live for twenty to thirty years before they develop any symptoms of the disease. Therefore, many arc unaware that they have the disease and don't get treatment for it. Without treatment, hepatitis gradually destroys the liver. Reed had long suffered from hepatitis. After his health rapidly declined in 2013, he received a liver transplant but never fully recovered.

The term hepatitis is used to describe anything that causes inflammation of the liver. It can be **acute** (lasting

Influential musician Lou Reed died of liver failure brought on by hepatitis C despite getting a transplant.

less than six months) or **chronic** (lasting more than six months). Hepatitis does not get the same attention as other deadly diseases, such as acquired immune deficiency syndrome (AIDS) and Ebola. This is understandable. Ebola is highly contagious and it kills quickly; the images of suffering around the world are horrible. AIDS has affected many people in the United States, some of them famous, and it continues to spread in the developing world.

However, the number of people worldwide suffering from one of the five forms of hepatitis is shocking. Reed's death alerted people to the scope of the problem. According to the Centers for Disease Control and Prevention (CDC), there were nearly four hundred million people living with chronic viral hepatitis in 2014. That is approximately one out of every twelve persons worldwide. These are the known cases, but the totals could be much higher. Many people blame the flu or other illnesses for their symptoms when they are really suffering from hepatitis.

One million deaths occur worldwide every year from complications due to hepatitis. Most of the deaths are related to **cirrhosis** or liver cancer.

All types of hepatitis eventually attack the liver, which filters toxins and waste from the blood and manages levels of cholesterol and hormones. Hepatitis is treatable. Most important, it is a disease that can often be avoided by taking certain precautions.

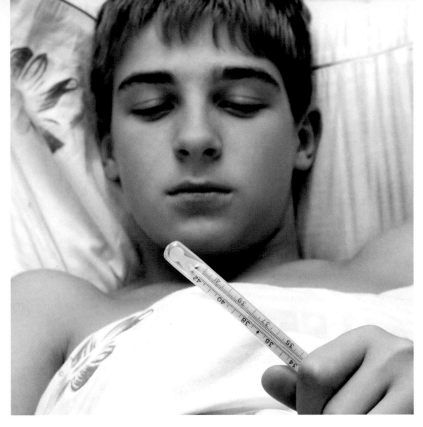
Hepatitis is often mistaken for the flu because they share some symptoms, including a fever.

Knowing about hepatitis and how to prevent it is the best way of avoiding the disease and stopping this silent epidemic in its tracks.

Reed had admitted to heavy drug use and said he used heroin and other drugs just to feel normal. He expected that despite years of carrying an infection a liver transplant would save him and that he would soon return to touring and performing concerts. This was not to be. He had overcome his addictions, but the disease had taken too heavy a toll on his body.

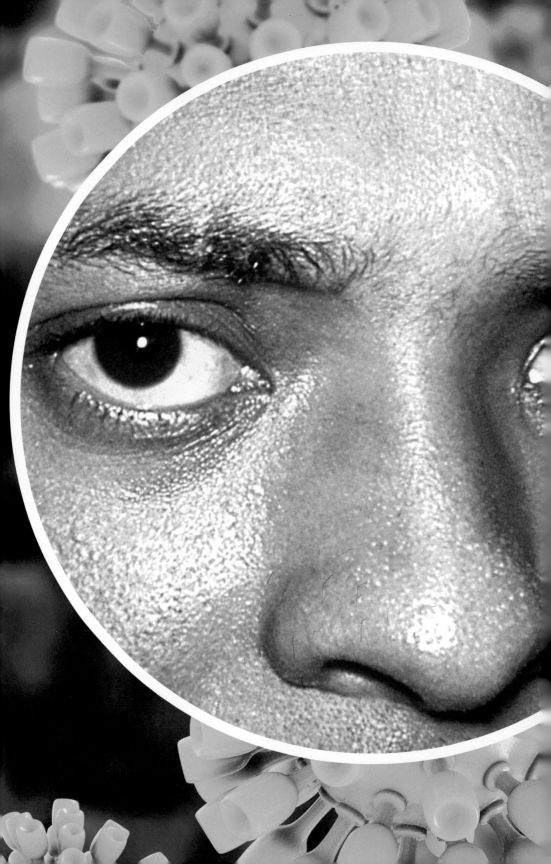

one Hidden for Centuries

There is one symptom that can point to the existence of hepatitis and other liver problems in a person, and it has been known for thousands of years. The visible symptom is **jaundice**, a yellowing of the skin or the whites of the eyes. According to the medical journal *Clinical Microbiology Review*, epidemic jaundice appeared in ancient Greece and Rome. The ancient Chinese were also aware of its existence.

There is a reference to jaundice in the Babylonian Talmud of the fifth century BCE and another in a letter from Pope Zacharias to St. Boniface in the eighth century CE. The first modern record of epidemic jaundice is from an **outbreak** on the Mediterranean island of Minorca in 1745. While scientists do not know for sure if this jaundice indicated a hepatitis outbreak, there was certainly a contagious disease on Minorca that affected the liver. There was another outbreak recorded in Germany in 1791.

The most visible symptom of hepatitis is jaundice, a yellowing of the skin or the eyes.

Many of the outbreaks of jaundice are associated with wars. During the Civil War, the Union Army reported 71,691 cases. Hepatitis is spread through **contaminated** food or water, or by contact with tainted blood. In Civil War field hospitals, surgical instruments were rarely sterilized between uses.

Although doctors did not have a name for hepatitis at this time, they learned a lot about the virus from studying outbreaks. By the early 1900s, doctors had learned that hepatitis passed from person to person through food, and possibly water.

H. C. Brown was a scientist who studied the 1931 jaundice outbreaks in England. He determined that jaundice was caused by an "ultra-microscopic virus" that appeared only in humans. Brown himself developed symptoms less than five weeks after handling samples from an outbreak in Yorkshire. This time span between infection and showing symptoms was the first hint doctors had about the actual **incubation** period of hepatitis.

According to the army's US Office of Medical History, there was an epidemic among American troops in 1942, and two hundred thousand cases among US soldiers between 1942 and 1945.

Human Guinea Pigs

Conscientious objectors faced a dilemma during World War II. They refused to fight on religious or humanitarian grounds, but they did not want to be

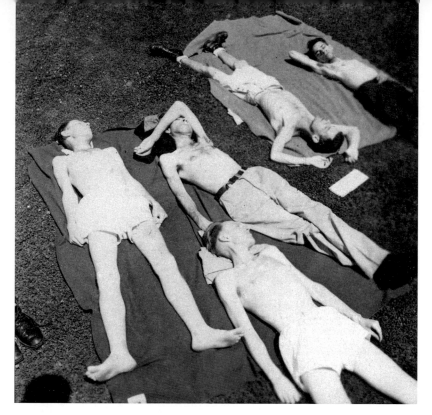

Conscientious objectors volunteered for tests during World War II, including one on the effects of starvation.

labeled as cowards when many others were sacrificing so much. They wanted to help the war effort in some way without killing.

In response, the United States developed the Civilian Public Service. The people involved fought forest fires, planted trees, and rebuilt roads. As many as five hundred civilians volunteered for medical experiments carried out by the US Office of Scientific Research and Development and the US Office of the Surgeon General. Some tests required them to suffer malnutrition, be covered in lice, and then be sprayed with the chemical DDT. In others, men were exposed to deadly diseases. In one test, men were inoculated with a hepatitis virus. From the tests, doctors learned more about the virus's incubation period and how it spread. About the tests, conscientious objector Neil Hartman said in a PBS documentary titled *The Good War and Those Who Refused to Fight It*:

> We were very concerned of course that we had been called all kinds of names, yellow bellies, and things like that. I had volunteered for an ambulance driver and got turned down. American Field Service, they said they didn't want any more COs, they had too many, but I was young and I wanted to show that I was not a coward, so when they offered me this chance of being a guinea pig, it fit right in with my scheme of things of proving that I was willing to take risks on my own body, but I just did not want to kill someone else.

The late Dr. C. Everett Koop, the US Surgeon General from 1981 to 1989, was a medical resident during these experiments. In that same documentary Koop said that he performed biopsies to determine how the virus affected the liver, including two on Hartman. He also learned that the men he examined had no idea that they could die during the experiments, which made it hard for him to be a part of the program.

"It couldn't happen today," Dr. Koop told PBS. "Internal Review Boards would not permit the use

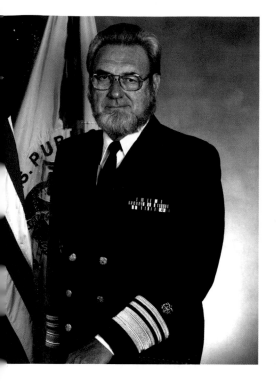

Dr. C. Everett Koop monitored hepatitis volunteers as a medical resident.

of a live virus in human subjects unless they really understood what was going to happen to them. And I doubt that even if they knew what the risk was, that an Internal Review Board in any academic institution would consent to that kind of experimental work."

Educated Guess

We can only speculate about how many of the historical cases of jaundice were actually hepatitis. The disease is caused by a virus, a small infectious microorganism that grows only inside the cells of other organisms. A virus is made of either deoxyribonucleic acid (DNA) or ribonucleic acid (RNA), the materials that make up genes. A virus is not alive and depends on other cells to spread throughout the body in a form called a virion. A virion is a virus particle made up of a protein shell covering a DNA or RNA core. When a virion enters the body, it is attracted to specific cells. The hepatitis virus is drawn to liver cells.

A Closer History

2000 BCE First recorded references to jaundice and other hepatitis symptoms.

1947 F. O. MacCallum identifies and names hepatitis A (spread by food and water) and hepatitis B (spread by blood).

1963 Baruch Blumberg and Harvey Alter discover the Aa antigen (later called HBsAg), later linked to hepatitis.

1968 Kazuo Okochi's experiments confirm that hepatitis is a virus and hepatitis B is spread through blood.

1970 D.S. Dane discovers the virion of the hepatitis B virus, and names it the Dane particle.

1971 Saul Krugman accidentally discovers that heating blood infected with hepatitis B could kill the virus.

1972 The United States requires all donated blood to be tested for hepatitis B.

1973–1974 Stephen Feinstone and Maurice Hilleman identify and describe the hepatitis A virus.

1978 Mario Rizzetto identifies hepatitis D.

1981 A hepatitis B vaccine developed by Hilleman is approved for public use.

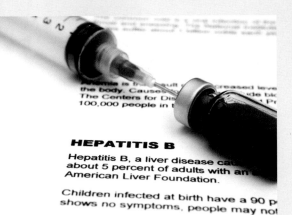

HEPATITIS B

Hepatitis B, a liver disease ca...
about 5 percent of adults with an...
American Liver Foundation.

Children infected at birth have a 90 p...
shows no symptoms, people may no...

A vaccine for hepatitis B was approved in 1981.

1983 Mikhail Balayan identifies hepatitis E.

1990 Tests are developed to find hepatitis C in blood.

1996 Hilleman develops a hepatitis A vaccine.

1997 Schering-Plough, Inc. introduces Intron A, the first **interferon** treatment for hepatitis C.

2011 Protease inhibitors Boceprevir and Telprevir, when combined with peg-interferon and ribavirin, increase cure rates of hepatitis C by 67 to 75 percent. Chronic hepatitis E is cured by ribavirin in trials.

July 2012 WHO releases Framework for Global Action, which describes areas to prevent, treat, and save lives of hepatitis victims.

December 2013 The Food and Drug Administration approves sofosbuvir, which treats hepatitis C without side effects.

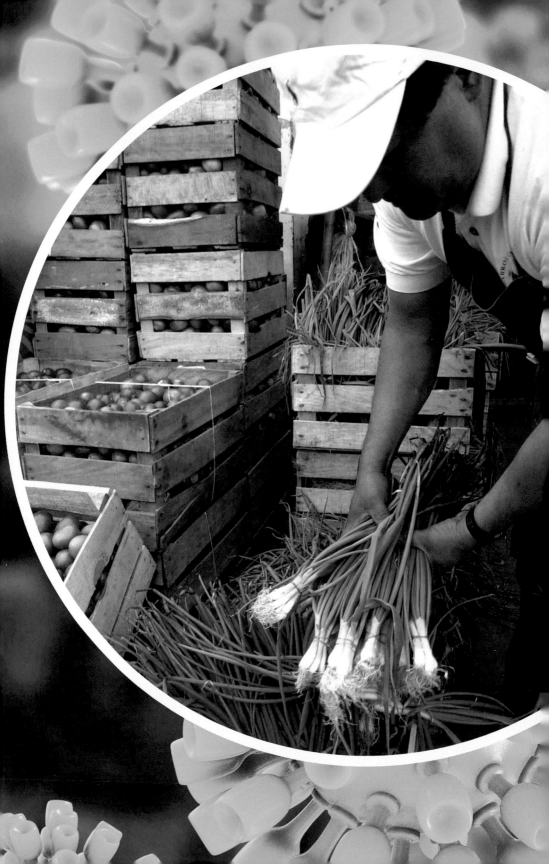

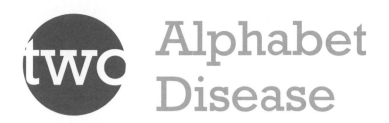

Alphabet Disease

two

A large outbreak of hepatitis A in 2013 was traced to health food. The Centers for Disease Control and Prevention confirmed that 165 people contracted the disease from eating an organic antioxidant blend sold by a large national retail chain.

The strain of the virus that sickened the people is found rarely in North America. It circulates mainly in North Africa and the Middle East. The source of the virus was determined to be pomegranate seeds imported from Turkey.

The disease hit people from late March through the middle of August of that year. Among those who became ill, sixty-nine were hospitalized but no deaths were reported. All of the products containing the pomegranate seeds were recalled and the outbreak was stopped.

Tainted green onions caused the largest hepatitis A outbreak ever in the United States.

In 2014, Health Care of Nevada (HCN) settled a lawsuit that was filed following an outbreak of hepatitis C. The disease was contracted at endoscopy clinics in HCN's network. A doctor who owned the clinics was convicted of twenty-seven criminal counts connected to the outbreak, including one for second-degree murder in the death of a seventy-seven-year-old woman.

Tainted green onions served at a Mexican restaurant in Monaca, Pennsylvania, caused the worst outbreak of hepatitis A in America. On October 5, 2003, John Spratt and his teenage daughter shared a plate of chicken fajitas at that restaurant. In the weeks that followed, Spratt felt as if he had a flu virus that wouldn't go away.

When the symptoms worsened, and Spratt could no longer keep any food or water down, he was hospitalized and treated for **dehydration**. "And then he unexpectedly went into liver failure," Spratt's brother, Joseph, told the *Pittsburgh Post-Gazette*. Spratt was admitted to the hospital on November 5. His doctors wanted to give him an immediate liver transplant, but Spratt never recovered long enough to sustain the surgery. He died on November 14, 2003, a victim of one of the largest hepatitis A outbreaks in the country.

Spratt was one of four victims of the outbreak who died of hepatitis A. The Pennsylvania Department of Health first learned about the outbreak in early November. It opened clinics and asked everyone who had eaten at the restaurant to be screened, or tested, for hepatitis A. About 10,000 people were screened, and 660 tested positive for hepatitis A, according to an Associated Press report in March 2004. Those who did not test positive were given an injection of immune globulin, a drug to keep them from getting the disease.

The outbreak was eventually traced to tainted green onions that had been imported from Mexico by the restaurant chain. The Associated Press reported on November 22, 2003, that the onions could have been contaminated in several ways, possibly from a sewage leak in a farmer's field or an unwashed truck that hauled the produce.

People contract hepatitis A from coming into contact with the **feces** of an infected person or from eating contaminated food. Most often, people who do not wash their hands after using the bathroom spread hepatitis A. For example, there is a restaurant in New Jersey that received multiple health violations in the months prior to an employee and many customers contracting hepatitis A in late 2014. An inspection report said employees at the restaurant regularly broke the health code of ethics, which involved separating raw foods, hand washing, proper sanitation, and preventing contamination. Cooking food usually kills the virus but the ingredients in salads and other raw foods can sicken people.

Not all forms of hepatitis are spread through poor hygiene or contaminated food. Following is a review of the different strains of hepatitis.

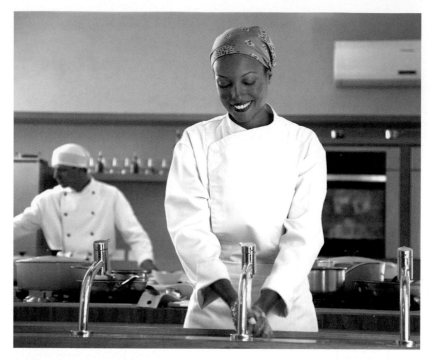

Restaurant workers should wash their hands carefully to avoid spreading hepatitis A.

Hepatitis A

Hepatitis A is rare in the United States and other wealthy nations because it is easier for people to practice good hygiene. Sewage is treated and contained, and not allowed to run into streets or fields where it could touch food. Garbage containers filled with dirty diapers or contaminated food is not kept in places where people live. Hot running water makes keeping clean easier, too.

What makes spreading hepatitis A, or HAV, even easier is that people often don't know they are infected.

People with hepatitis A can feel tired or nauseous, have fevers, lose their appetites, or have a stomachache. In some cases, the patient will have jaundice. He or she may also expel urine that seems darker than normal. In many cases, hepatitis A tends to incubate for about thirty days before symptoms appear. After the incubation period, an infected person experiences nausea, vomiting, abdominal pain, and a decreased appetite. Jaundice, itching, and darkened urine appear about two weeks later, as initial symptoms decrease.

For the most part, HAV feels a lot like the flu. The symptoms last less than two months for most people and the infection is gone. Since HAV can only be **diagnosed** with a blood test, many are unknowingly infected.

Hepatitis has an incubation period in the body of about twenty-eight days. This means the disease only survives in the body for that long, and can only be spread during that time. However, the CDC says twenty-eight days is not an absolute number. To be certain that one is without disease, the incubation range is fifteen to fifty days.

There are two vaccines for hepatitis A. Because the disease is so rare in the United States, the vaccine is only given to someone at risk of contracting the disease. For instance, if someone were going to visit a country with poor sanitation and hygiene, he or she would likely get the vaccine before their trip. (According to the CDC, Mexico, Bolivia, Paraguay, much of the Middle East, and nearly all of Africa have high rates of hepatitis A.) However, if a person is exposed to hepatitis A, he or she can be injected with immune globulin to prevent infection. In order for the immune globulin to work, the person must be injected with it within two weeks of exposure to hepatitis A. Only in very few cases does hepatitis A continue to cause problems after the initial, acute infection. Medically, acute means "having a rapid onset and following a short but severe course." The hepatitis A virus does not typically cause long-term damage to the liver.

Hepatitis B

The CDC estimates that 18,800 people were infected with hepatitis B in 2011, and that 1,792 died from it in 2010. Today, up to 1.4 million people in the United States have chronic cases of HBV. The number of cases has dropped dramatically from the mid-1980s, when there were about 27,000 new cases reported annually.

The virus is spread by coming into contact with the blood or bodily fluids of an infected person. Sharing intravenous needles and having unprotected sex with infected people are the most common ways of contracting hepatitis B, or HBV, which is easier to contract than the human immunodeficiency virus (HIV). The virus is not spread through casual contact, such as shaking hands with or hugging an infected person.

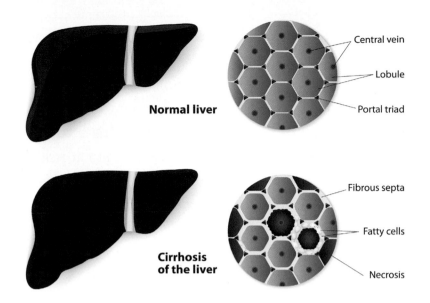

Normal liver

Central vein

Lobule

Portal triad

Cirrhosis of the liver

Fibrous septa

Fatty cells

Necrosis

Cirrhosis changes the structure of the liver.

As with hepatitis A, it is possible to have hepatitis B and not know it. Only a blood test can confirm if someone has the virus. The symptoms for HAV and HBV can be similar, too. Infected people can feel flu-like symptoms, such as joint pain or fever. Hepatitis B can also cause extreme fatigue. At times, people with HBV are unable to get out of bed and go about their day for weeks or months.

There are several treatment options for chronic hepatitis B. Included are antivirals, interferons, and nucleoside reverse transcriptase inhibitors (NRTIs) that slow the ability of the virus to multiply. An interferon is a **synthetic** copy of a protein the immune system produces to fight infection. Common side effects connected with interferons include fatigue, muscle aches and headaches, fever, and hair loss. These treatments do not cure the disease, but they do suppress it.

About 90 to 95 percent of people infected with acute HBV recover fully and are immune to the virus for the rest of their lives. The remaining 5 to 10 percent become carriers of the disease and are at risk for developing chronic infections. Older HBV patients sometimes develop chronic liver disease, such as cirrhosis. This happens when hardened fibers (fibrosis) develop in the liver. This scar tissue can block the flow of blood through the liver and affect its function. It is a condition often associated with alcoholism.

Hepatitis C

Hepatitis C can only be spread through blood. Some people get hepatitis C (HCV) from sharing intravenous needles. Others have the virus because they received blood or organs from an infected person. Although HCV can be spread through unprotected sexual contact, contracting the disease in this way is rare. Sharing eating utensils or drinks, hugging, or being sneezed or coughed on by an infected person cannot spread the disease. People with HCV are at little risk of infecting those with whom they live, work, or attend school.

Hepatitis C sometimes causes flu-like symptoms similar to those of HAV and HBV, but may be asymptomatic, which means that it shows no symptoms at all. However, chronic hepatitis C can do more significant liver damage than other types of hepatitis. Of every one hundred people who have HCV, seventy-five to eighty-five of them may develop long-term, or chronic, infections, and seventy may develop chronic liver disease. Another fifteen of those one hundred people infected could, over twenty to thirty years, develop cirrhosis of the liver. Because HCV is so damaging to the liver, people with the disease are often candidates for liver transplants.

Variations of HCV, called hepatitis G and GB virus C, were discovered in 1996. It is carried in the blood and causes a persistent infection for up to nine years in 15 to 30 percent of adults. There is no treatment for this virus, and very little is known about it.

Hepatitis D and Hepatitis E

People with hepatitis D (also called the delta virus) cannot have it without also having hepatitis B. Hepatitis D (HDV) is an "incomplete" virus. In order to contract HDV, a person needs to already be infected with HBV. Having HBV does not automatically mean someone will also get HDV. The hepatitis D symptoms are similar to those of hepatitis B, though HDV can cause more severe liver damage than HBV.

Hepatitis E (HEV) is similar to hepatitis A in that it is mainly transmitted by drinking water contaminated by diseased fecal matter. Unlike HAV, it is rare for HEV to be passed from person to person by food or touch.

Mother to Child

When a mother transmits hepatitis to her child, it is usually hepatitis B. There are fifteen thousand women with hepatitis B who give birth in the United States each year. Some show no symptoms, so the CDC recommends that all women get screened for the disease during their first prenatal visit.

This disease is highly contagious, and is commonly passed on during delivery, when the child is exposed to blood and fluids that can carry the virus. Doctors take steps to protect both mother and child when a pregnant woman is diagnosed with hepatitis B. The mother will receive HBV immune globulin. The newborn will be given the HBV immune globulin at birth, and three subsequent doses until he or she is six months of age. This cuts the rate of infection in the newborn from 0 to 3 percent.

There is one further danger to the child. If an infected woman is being treated with Rebetron, a combination therapy, she should not breastfeed her child. Scientists don't know what adverse effects the child might suffer from digesting breast milk containing the drugs.

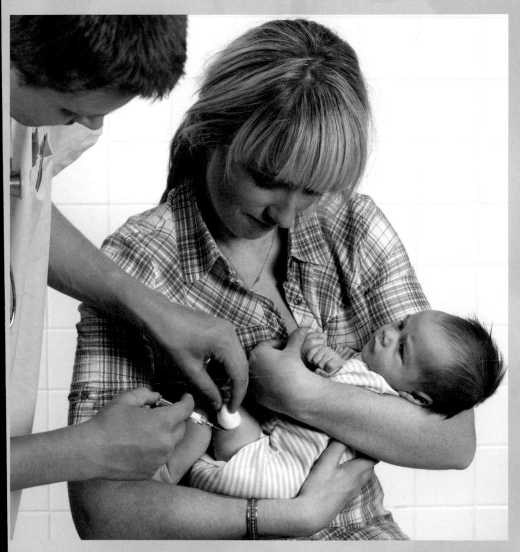

A series of inoculations are given to a child whose mother has hepatitis B.

Nearly all reported cases of HEV in the United States occur in people exposed to the virus in countries with poor sanitary conditions.

Hepatitis E is less likely to cause infection than HAV. Although the virus has a low fatality rate (1 percent), women, especially pregnant women, are at a much greater risk of dying from hepatitis E.

Twin Killers

Unprotected sex and injecting drugs intravenously are among the risky behaviors that spread hepatitis B and hepatitis C. These are the same behaviors that spread the human immunodeficiency virus, or HIV. HIV is the virus that causes AIDS, or acquired immunodeficiency syndrome.

According to the website aids.gov, more than one-third of people infected with HIV are also infected with HBV (10 percent) and HCV (25 percent). HIV weakens the immune system. This leaves people co-infected with hepatitis more likely to suffer liver-related health problems.

People with HIV and hepatitis infections are at increased risk of life-threatening complications. Those who are co-infected with hepatitis C and HIV should be vaccinated against hepatitis A and B. And anyone with HIV should be tested for HBV and HCV. Antiretroviral drugs have allowed people with HIV to

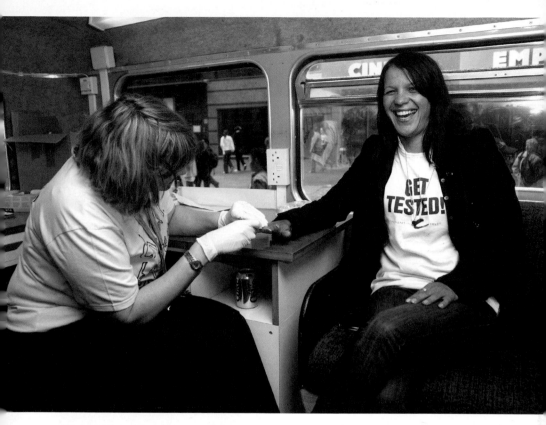

People should get tested for hepatitis if there is any chance they might have been exposed.

live longer, but liver disease has become the leading cause of non-AIDS-related deaths in this group.

HIV and hepatitis are both viruses and can only be treated with vaccines. Antibiotics won't work against any virus. They can be used only to treat infections caused by bacteria. Common bacterial infections include pneumonia, ear infections, and skin disorders.

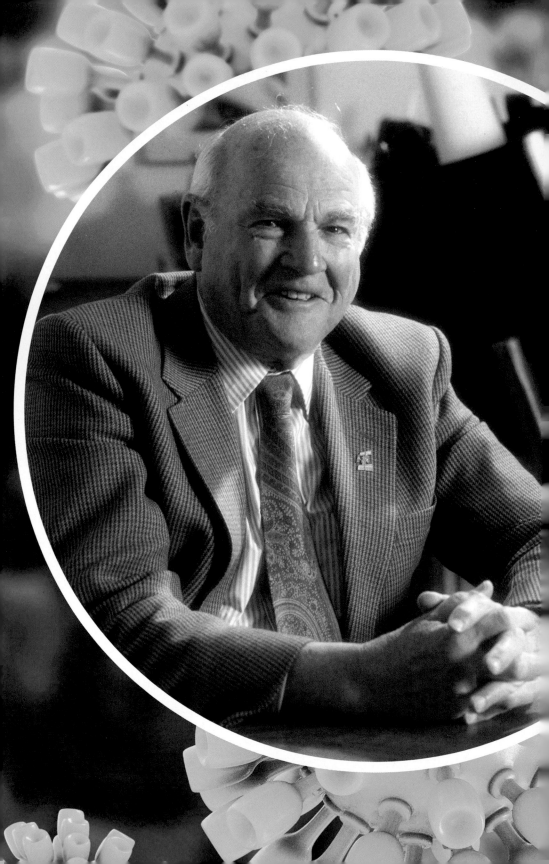

three A Long Process

Doctors can now treat hepatitis B, which is the main cause of liver cancer worldwide, but they can't cure it. Their big breakthrough in treatment came, as in Dr. MacCallum's case, from a scientist who wasn't even studying the disease.

Dr. Baruch Blumberg wanted to know why some people were more susceptible to diseases than others. He traveled the world collecting blood samples. Working with another scientist named Harvey Alter from the National Institutes of Health blood bank, Dr. Blumberg found, in 1963, an antigen that is rarely present in the blood of healthy people. An antigen is something foreign to the body that causes a reaction from the body's immune system. The antigen was present in people who received several blood transfusions, such as hemophiliacs. Blumberg and Alter named the antigen Aa, or Australian antigen, because one blood sample they studied came from an

The work of Dr. Baruch Blumberg, shown here in 1999, led to the vaccine for hepatitis B.

aboriginal person from Australia. The antigen is now called HBsAg.

Scientists began testing for HBsAg in people with leukemia to determine if the antigen was one of the causes for the disease. In 1966, Blumberg, W. Thomas London, and Alton Sutnik discovered that a twelve-year-old boy acquired HBsAg months after he had tested negative for the antigen. During that time, the boy was also diagnosed with hepatitis. It seemed that HBsAg was linked to hepatitis. The link made even more sense after Blumberg's lab technician came down with hepatitis. She tested her own blood for HBsAg— the result was positive. The technician became one of the first people diagnosed with hepatitis through the HBsAg test.

While scientists all over the world were researching the HBsAg link to hepatitis B, Dr. Alfred Prince at the New York Blood Center took blood samples from several patients who received multiple transfusions. In 1968, one of Prince's patients began showing symptoms of hepatitis. In the early samples of the man's blood, there was no HBsAg. After the patient started feeling ill, however, blood tests revealed the presence of HBsAg.

Also in 1968, at the University of Tokyo in Japan, a scientist named Kazuo Okochi found that blood that tested positive for HBsAg was much more likely to transmit hepatitis to patients than blood that tested negative. In 1970, doctors at Middlesex Hospital in London saw virus particles in the blood of people with HBsAg. They also saw the virus in liver cells of patients with hepatitis. These discoveries confirmed much of what scientists had been thinking for years. Hepatitis was a virus and, in the case of hepatitis B, it was passed through the blood.

In 1971, Saul Krugman, an infectious disease specialist at New York University, made an accidental discovery. Krugman learned that samples of HBV-contaminated blood that had been heated to kill viruses gave some protection against the spread of the disease. Blumberg, then at Fox Chase Cancer Center in Philadelphia, Pennsylvania, thought that a vaccine could be made from particles of HBsAg.

Blumberg's idea was unique. Previously, vaccines had only been made from weakened strains of a virus or from different viruses that were similar to those being vaccinated against. Also, vaccines could be made from whole viruses or bacteria that were killed using heat or cold to prevent infection.

What Dr. Blumberg proposed was using only little pieces, or subunits, of a virus. Maurice Hilleman at the Merck Institute for Science Education thought Dr. Blumberg had the right idea. With permission from Fox Chase, Hilleman, in 1971, began work on using subunits to make a vaccine. It was not until 1980 that the Merck team created a vaccine that was 90 percent

Testing Blood Supply

There are many groups at high risk for contracting HCV. One has been eliminated: people who need blood transfusions.

There was no way to test donated blood for the presence of HCV before 1990. Because of this, the rate of transmission of the disease was 8 to 10 percent among people who received blood. Among hemophiliacs, who often receive transfusions, the infection rate was as high as 40 percent. Women who underwent a Cesarean section were also infected at a high rate, as this procedure often required blood transfusions.

Once tests for HCV in the blood supply were discovered, the infection rate from medical procedures dropped. By 1993, the rate fell to about 1 percent, and today it has fallen to almost 0 percent. Blood banks now inform any donor whose blood tests positive for hepatitis.

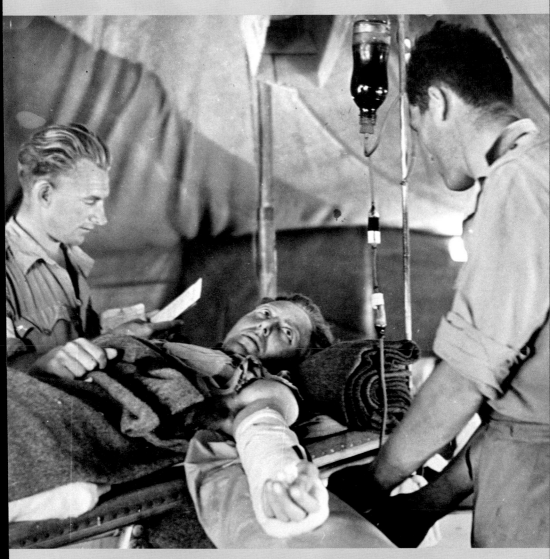

Soldiers given blood transfusions in field hospitals in the mid-twentieth century could be exposed to hepatitis C.

effective against HBV and, most important, had no adverse side effects. The vaccine, which was called heptavax, was made available to the public in 1981.

The complication involved in producing the vaccine was that it required large amounts of hepatitis B–infected blood. However, in 1977, William Rutter at the University of California, San Francisco, solved the problem. Rutter learned how to make the virus automatically replicate itself in a process called recombinant technology. Not only could large batches of the vaccine be produced, there would be no danger of the vaccine containing blood tainted with other diseases.

The research into HBV encouraged other scientists to learn more about the other forms of hepatitis. In 1973, scientists at the National Institutes of Health used an electron microscope to view the hepatitis A virus in human **stools** for the first time. Hilleman used his work from HBV to find a vaccine for HAV. In 1996, Hilleman developed a vaccine made from a modified version of the hepatitis A virus. Tests to determine the presence of HCV in the blood were not developed until 1990.

Hepatitis D—which depends on hepatitis B to survive—was discovered in 1978 by an Italian scientist named Mario Rizzetto. Hepatitis E was not discovered until 1983, when Russian scientist, Mikhail Balayan noticed a new type of hepatitis virus in localized epidemics, also spread by contaminated water.

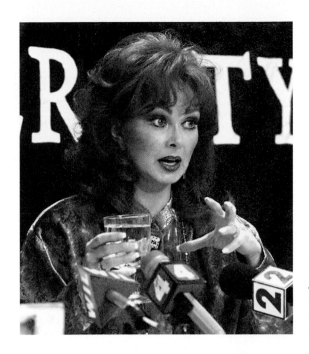

Singer Naomi Judd contracted hepatitis C when she worked as a nurse.

Advances in the treatment of HCV came just in time to help singer Naomi Judd. She became famous as one-half of the mother-daughter country duo the Judds. In a seven-year span, the Judds had twenty Top Ten hit songs, and Naomi won a Grammy Award for writing "Love Can Build a Bridge." In 1991, the duo stopped performing because Naomi had contracted HCV and was told she had only three years to live. Naomi believes she got HCV in the early 1980s, from a needle stick when she was working as an intensive care unit nurse. She began interferon treatment, injecting the medicine into her abdomen. It made her feel depressed and as if she had the flu. Doctors balanced the side effects with the antidepressant drug Zoloft.

The medication worked and Naomi is now HCV free. In 1991, she created the Naomi Judd Education and Research Fund to educate people about hepatitis. The fund also raises money for the American Liver Foundation (ALF), the organization for which Naomi serves as spokesperson.

Early Treatment

People diagnosed with hepatitis C are usually treated with a combination of drugs. The treatment can last twelve to twenty-four weeks. Patients are considered

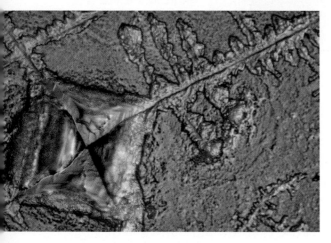

cured of HCV when they have what is called a sustained virologic response. This means the virus is undetectable twelve to twenty-four weeks after treatment ends.

This interferon protein was produced in response to a viral infection.

Interferon therapy was the first reliable way to cure HCV. Interferon is a natural substance that was discovered in 1957. Cells infected with a virus secrete a material that prevents other cells around it from being infected. Scientists called the material interferon because it "interfered" with the natural replication of the virus in the body.

The pharmaceutical company Schering-Plough, Inc. created the drug Intron A, the first interferon therapy. The Food and Drug Administration (FDA), the government agency that regulates drugs, approved Intron A for use for hepatitis in 1997. Interferon therapy can prevent further damage to the liver and suppresses the virus enough so it can no longer be detected in the blood.

In June 1998, the FDA approved interferon alpha plus ribavirin, or Rebetron. Ribavirin also boosts the body's immune system and helps interferons prevent the replication of the virus.

Interferon therapy can also have side effects. The most common complaint among those undergoing interferon therapy is that they experience flu-like symptoms. Since the body reacts to the flu by sending out interferon to fight the virus, it makes sense that elevated levels of interferon in the body can feel the same way. In a few cases, people feel depressed or lose their hair in reaction to interferon. Doctors monitor such side effects and often can control them by changing the dose, or amount, of interferon a patient takes.

Doctors recognizing the difficulties associated with interferon treatment pushed on for other ways to battle the disease. They have made some exciting discoveries.

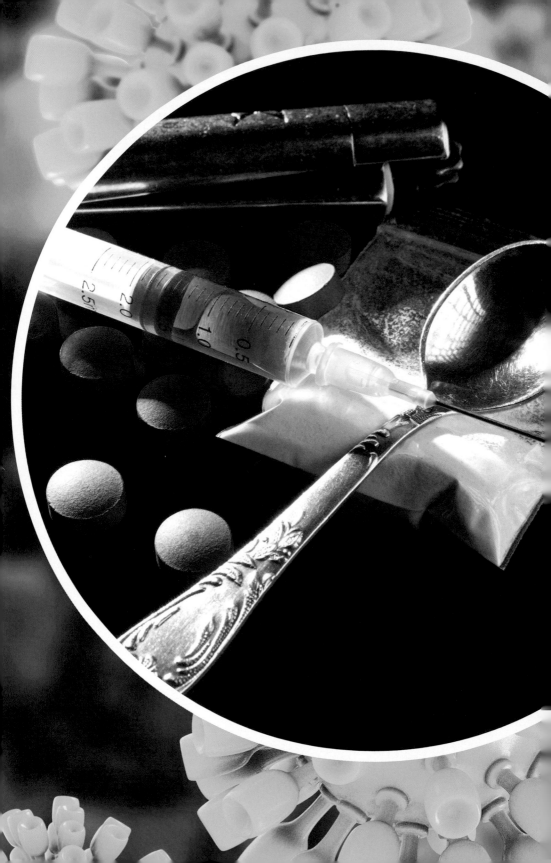

four Getting Younger

Hepatitis was considered a disease of the Baby Boomer generation. People of that age contracted the disease often before its causes were known. In 1993, people aged thirty to forty-nine had the highest incidence of hepatitis C.

However, after years of falling hepatitis infection rates in the United States, new infections are again on the rise. Also, the virus is showing up in the youth of this country. Most of the people with new infections are between the ages of twenty and twenty-nine, and the number of cases of acute HCV among those younger than nineteen has doubled. There was a 200 percent increase in acute infections in people under the age of thirty in a majority of the states between 2006 and 2012.

The primary reason is an increase in intravenous drug use, and it is tied to the growing problem of prescription drug abuse. Oxycodone is a commonly

Cases of hepatitis C are on the rise among younger drug users from the suburbs.

Risky Behaviors

Actress Pamela Anderson has hepatitis C, and she claims she contracted the disease from her former husband, rock drummer Tommy Lee. She admitted in an interview that they each got a tattoo from an artist who used the same needle on the two of them. She added that Lee already had the disease and didn't tell her. Lee argues that Anderson's account is untrue.

However, getting a tattoo is a common way to contract hepatitis C. Even if the tattoo artist changes and sterilizes the needles between uses, the virus can seep into the ink and be spread. Other skin-piercing practices, such as body piercing and acupuncture, have also increased the incidence of hepatitis C. The largest factor in the spread of the disease, however, is intravenous drug use.

Cocaine users can also pass on the disease as straws used to snort the drug can become infected. Promiscuous sexual behavior is another primary cause, with active homosexuals bearing the greatest risk. Prison populations are also high risk, with some institutions reporting rates of nearly 100 percent.

According to the website epidemic.org, "The primary risk factors for infection being greater numbers of partners, unprotected sex, simultaneous infection with other STDs, and traumatic sexual activity."

prescribed and abused painkiller. It is a narcotic and highly addictive. People who become addicted often turn to crushing oxycodone pills, dissolving the powder in water, and injecting it to get high more quickly. This can lead to the use of heroin, which can be less expensive. Sharing needles while injecting drugs spreads hepatitis.

More than three-quarters of the new HCV infections reported among today's youth are spread by drug injection. The youth who get sick are overwhelmingly white, and more than half come from suburban or rural areas. Seventy-six percent said they tried a prescription drug before injecting a drug. More than half of all intravenous drug users now contract HCV.

When people think of an epidemic, they probably think of AIDS or the black plague. Those are traditional epidemics, diseases that spread rapidly and affect many individuals in a specific location. Hepatitis, because it can be transmitted in different ways and often does not kill people, is a disease not often considered an epidemic.

It is easy to assume that like AIDS, hepatitis spreads rapidly and is considered an outbreak. An outbreak of hepatitis A, such as the one in Pittsburgh, hits many people at once. But in most instances, these people recover. It is unlikely that a hepatitis A outbreak will result in the deaths of thousands of people, as did the plague outbreak. Hepatitis B is, for most people, a one-time infection. Although the disease can become chronic, a good portion of those who are infected with hepatitis B will recover. In addition, vaccinations against hepatitis A and B help keep the disease from spreading in the first place.

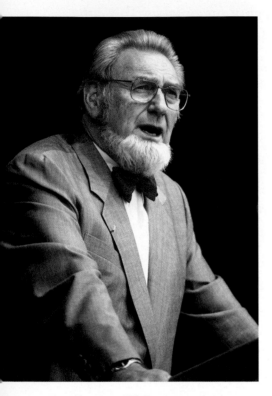

Former US Surgeon General C. Everett Koop was concerned with the spread of hepatitis C.

Hepatitis C, though, has the characteristics of an epidemic. The late C. Everett Koop, the former US surgeon general, explained that hepatitis C is "one of the most significant preventable and treatable public health problems facing our nation today."

According to the World Health Organization, 130 million to 150 million people globally have chronic hepatitis C infection, and 350,000 to 500,000 people die each year from liver diseases caused by the infection.

In 15 to 45 percent of all infected persons, the body clears itself of the virus spontaneously. The rest will develop chronic HCV infection. The risk of cirrhosis of the liver among those with a chronic infection is 15 to 30 percent within twenty years.

Hepatitis C infects three times as many people as AIDS, although people often suffer from both. One-third of all liver transplants performed in America are done on hepatitis C patients. Around the world, 75 percent of all liver disease is related to hepatitis C.

The body's immune system is better at overcoming hepatitis A and B than hepatitis C. Since the immune system tries so hard to fight the virus, people with hepatitis C often feel as though they have the flu. Flu-like symptoms will come and go over the years, so those who have HCV often don't even know they are sick. Not only does this make it easier for carriers to spread the virus, it makes it harder for them to be treated. Since people don't know they are sick, they won't seek the medical help that could prevent extensive liver damage. This is why some doctors refer to hepatitis C as "the silent epidemic."

There are many cases of infection that bear this out. Singer Gregg Allman, who founded the Allman Brothers Band, needed a liver transplant in 2010. The sixty-two-year-old said that he contracted hepatitis C at a tattoo parlor when he was twenty but wasn't diagnosed until 1999. Grammy-winning singer Natalie Cole was diagnosed with hepatitis C in 2008. She blamed her infection on her chronic drug use during the seventies.

Others who have battled the disease include Aerosmith's Steven Tyler, singer David Crosby, Anthony Kiedis of the Red Hot Chili Peppers, and

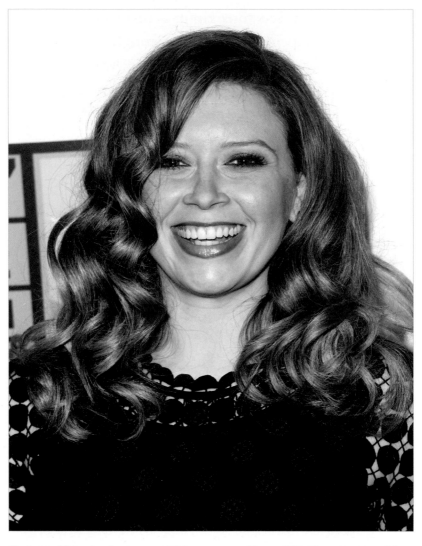

Actress Natasha Lyonne said her case of hepatitis C was caused by intravenous drug use.

Natasha Lyonne. Lyonne blamed her infection and subsequent medical problems on years of drug use. Since getting treatment, she has resumed her career and even landed a role on the popular television series *Orange Is the New Black*.

The late Dr. Koop was quoted: "We stand at the precipice of a grave threat to our public health. It affects people from all walks of life, in every state, in every country. And unless we do something about it soon, it will kill more people than AIDS."

For most people who contract hepatitis A or B, it is an acute, or short-term, infection. People infected with HAV or HBV become ill quickly. Their symptoms can be severe, but it is most often a one-time infection. With hepatitis C, and in some cases hepatitis B, the infection can be chronic. A chronic disease is one that causes a person to be ill for a long period of time. People with hepatitis C who go undiagnosed will deal with the disease for their entire lives. The virus could then do serious damage to the liver.

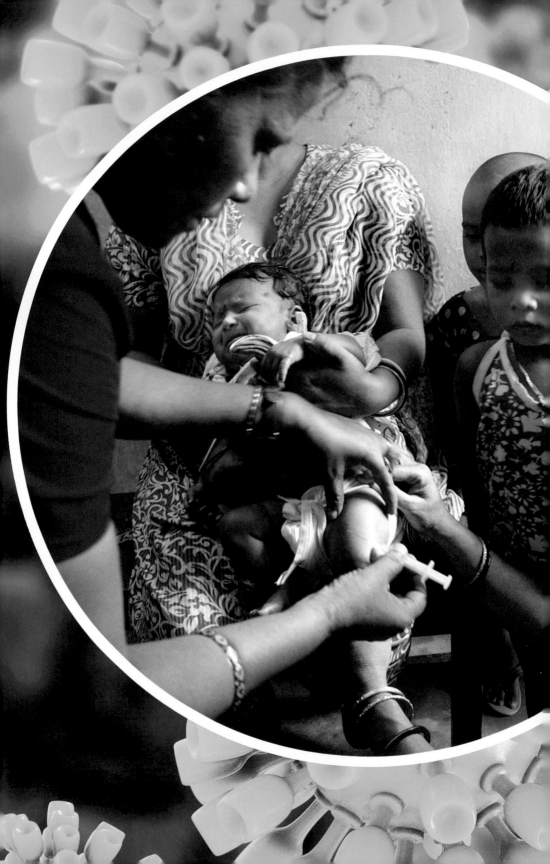

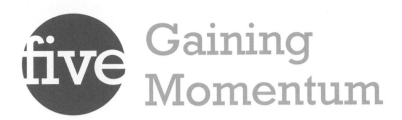

five Gaining Momentum

Medical science has made a lot of progress in the fight against all forms of hepatitis. There is now a vaccine for HAV and HBV. The vaccine makes 90 percent of the people infected immune to the disease, including infants. It doesn't work as well in people with compromised, or weakened, immune systems.

This vaccine has greatly reduced HBV infections in North America. Here is a partial list of people for whom the vaccine is recommended:

- All infants at birth, or children eighteen years old or younger who have not been vaccinated
- Sexually active people who are not in long-term, mutually monogamous relationships
- Men who have sex with men
- People living with HIV
- Injection drug users

All infants should receive the vaccination for hepatitis B.

- People with hepatitis C virus and other chronic liver diseases
- People with jobs in which there is a risk of infection (such as emergency medical technicians, doctors, and nurses)
- Travelers to regions with moderate or high rates of HBV infection
- **Hemodialysis** patients

There is no vaccine for HCV, but there are steps you can take to avoid getting it (these also work for avoiding HBV):

- Stop all injection drug use. If you choose to do so, be sure to use new, **sterile** syringes every time you inject. Never reuse or share anything used to prepare or inject drugs.
- Do not share toothbrushes or razors because they can be exposed to blood.
- Make sure that any tattoo or body piercing is performed by licensed experts who follow sterile procedures.

Doctors can recommend that people who are involved in risky behaviors get screened for hepatitis. However, patients don't often tell their doctors the truth about their behavior. Also, medical workers are often uncomfortable asking such personal questions.

People should not avoid hepatitis screening. Much progress has been made in treating the disease.

Scientists have found new ways to stop hepatitis B from replicating. The National Institutes of Health is funding research to expanding these discoveries into curing patients of the disease.

Liver cancer is increasing at a faster rate than any other cancer in the United States. Because hepatitis B causes most of the cases of liver cancer, curing people of hepatitis B would lower the incidence of this deadly condition.

Hepatitis C is a major cause of liver transplants, such as the one that the late Lou Reed underwent. These transplants don't cure people because the virus can damage the new liver.

Until recently, treatments for HCV involved interferons. The problem with interferons is their side effects, which is why scientists are so excited about a new hepatitis treatment that doesn't use them. In late 2013, the Food and Drug Administration approved the drug sofosbuvir, which had been synthesized six years earlier. The drug's brand name is Sovaldi.

One of the reasons many drugs cause problems in the body is that they don't work only on the region they are targeting. These drugs alter nucleosides, which are the building blocks of DNA and RNA. When the nucleosides are chemically changed they can stop chains of genetic code, and this can keep viruses inside cells from reproducing. However, these drugs don't enter the cells they are altering so they affect other areas of the body. This is what causes the side effects.

Ignorance Is Death

Not knowing if you have had hepatitis B can be very dangerous. In early 2015, a published study showed that chemotherapy and treatment with immunosuppressive medications can reactivate hepatitis B. Immunosuppressive drugs are used to treat leukemia, lymphoma, and transplant rejection. If hepatitis B is reactivated it can be severe, causing acute liver failure. One study showed that in 25 percent of cases when hepatitis B was reactivated, the patients died. This is why anyone about to undergo cancer treatments or an **organ transplant** should be screened for hepatitis B.

People receiving these treatments may be just a small part of the problem. Researchers also believe that the disease may be reactivated by medications used to treat things such as **rheumatoid arthritis**, the digestive conditions Crohn's and colitis, and skin conditions such as psoriasis.

One of the authors of the study, Dr. Adrian Di Bisceglie of Saint Louis University School of Medicine, said that HBV reactivation "may be an under-appreciated clinical challenge." He suggests further study and cooperation among medical disciplines to try to figure out the problems of HBV reactivation.

Michael Sofia developed sofosbuvir to attack the many forms of hepatitis C. His goal was to wrap his drug inside something he called an invisible cloak that would allow it to get into liver cells. Once there, the liver's enzymes would remove the cloak and the drug would be trapped inside the cell. That way, it could not escape to interact with other parts of the body and there would be no side effects.

"It does exactly what we designed it to do, which is one of those things that hardly ever happens," Sofia said during an interview with the *New Yorker*.

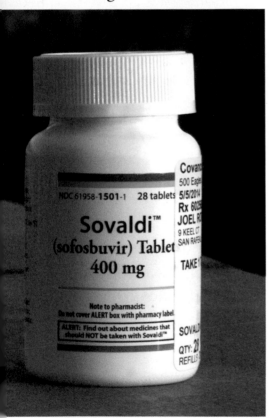

Sovaldi works against hepatitis C, but it is very expensive.

Sovaldi is in pill form and needs to be taken only once a day. It can be administered in very high doses. It works so well that Sofia is now working on a drug that targets hepatitis B. The drug company Gilead has run successful trials for an HBV drug.

The biggest problem with Sovaldi is its cost. In 2011, Gilead paid $11 billion for Pharmasset, the biotechnology firm that created the drug. Each pill costs $1,000, so treatment could be more

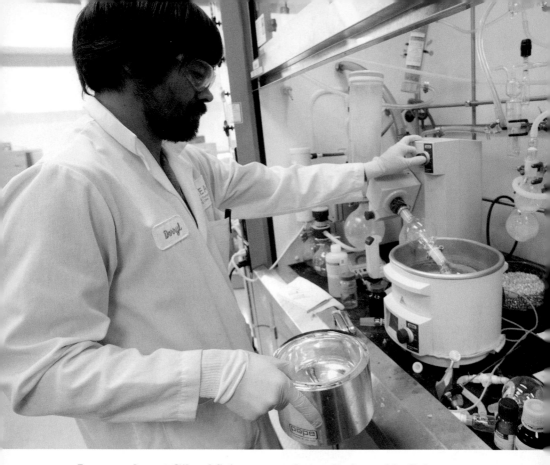

A researcher at Gilead Sciences works on the hepatitis C drug in 2012.

than $100,000 per patient. Other countries are upset at the price, reacting much the way they did when the first HIV drugs were introduced. For example, the National Health Service in the United Kingdom blocked the introduction of the medicine despite the fact that it was approved for use by the National Institute for Health and Care Excellence. That body approves drugs it considers cost-effective.

Sales of Sovaldi have been huge in the United States, but hepatitis is really a worldwide problem. The WHO reports that about 350 million people with HBV remain infected chronically. Seventy-five percent of people reside in areas where there are high levels of infection. One in four people with acute clinical cases of HBV, or one million people a year, die from chronic active hepatitis, cirrhosis, or primary liver cancer.

Globally, the most common way of passing on the disease is through childbirth. If the mother is an HBV carrier and is HBsAg-positive, her newborn has a 90 percent chance of becoming infected. Children can be protected from HBV if they receive the vaccine at birth. If they don't get the vaccine, they are likely to develop lifelong HBV infections that lead to liver failure or cancer.

Until effective vaccines can be developed against all forms of the disease and then distributed to all corners of the globe, hepatitis will remain a silent killer.

Glossary

acute Having a sudden onset, sharp rise, and short course.

chronic An illness that recurs or is experienced over a long period of time.

cirrhosis A chronic liver disease distinguished by degeneration of cells, inflammation, and fibrous thickening of tissue.

contaminate To make (something) impure by exposure to, or addition of, a poisonous or polluting substance; to infect.

contract To catch or acquire, as in a disease.

dehydration The excessive loss of water from the body.

diagnose To identify the nature of a disease or condition in a person by examining the symptoms.

feces Human or animal solid waste.

hemodialysis Purification of the blood by dialysis when the kidney no longer works.

incubation The period of time starting from when a pathogen enters the body until symptoms appear.

interferon A protein released by animal cells—usually in response to the entry of a virus—that inhibits virus replication.

jaundice Yellowing of the skin or whites of the eyes; due to an excess of the pigment bilirubin caused by obstruction of the bile duct or by liver disease.

liver A large organ in the body that serves many functions, among them the removal of toxins from the blood.

organ transplant The surgical replacement of a diseased organ with a healthy one.

outbreak A sudden rise in the incidence of a disease especially to epidemic or near epidemic proportions.

rheumatoid arthritis A chronic, progressive disease that causes inflammation and pain in the joints.

sterile Clean or free from bacteria or other contamination.

stools A discharge of fecal matter.

synthetic Something that is not natural; made from combining substances.

For More Information

Hepatitis Magazine

www.hepmag.com

This website provides an easy-to-understand overview on the different forms of hepatitis and its treatment, prevention, and symptoms.

WebMD Hepatitis Health Center

www.webmd.com/hepatitis/understanding-hepatitis-basics

Get the basics on this deadly disease, from what it is to its causes.

World Health Organization Fact Sheets

www.who.int/mediacentre/factsheets/en

Search these fact sheets for information on the causes, treatments, and spread of diseases throughout the world. Included are separate pages for hepatitis A, B, C, and E.

Interested in learning more about hepatitis?
Check out these websites and organizations.

Organizations

American Liver Foundation
75 Maiden Lane, Suite 603
New York, NY 10038
(800) 465-4837
www.liverfoundation.org

Centers for Disease Control and Prevention (CDC)
1600 Clifton Road
Atlanta, GA 30333
(800) 311-3435
(800) 232-2522 (Immunization hotline)
www.cdc.gov

Hepatitis B Foundation
700 East Butler Avenue
Doylestown, PA 18901-2697
(215) 489-4900
www.hepb.org

Hepatitis Foundation International
504 Black Drive
Sliver Spring, MD 20904-2901
(800) 891-0707
www.hepfi.org

For Further Reading

Books

Friedlander, Mark P. Jr. *Outbreak: Disease Detectives at Work*. Discovery. Minneapolis, MN: Twenty-First Century Books, 2009.

Hayhurst, Chris. *Everything You Need to Know About Hepatitis C*. New York: The Rosen Publishing Group, Inc., 2003.

Kaplan, Rosalind. *The Patient in the White Coat: My Odyssey from Health to Sickness and Back*. New York: Kaplan Publishing, 2012.

McKnight, Evelyn V., and Travis T. Bennington. *A Never Event: Exposing the Largest Outbreak of Hepatitis C in American Healthcare History*. Palisades, NY: History Examined LLC, 2014.

Paul, Nina L. *Living With Hepatitis C for Dummies*. Hoboken, NJ: For Dummies, 2005.

Index

Page numbers in **boldface** are illustrations. Entries in **boldface** are glossary terms.

Index